ESSENTIAL
WHOLE BODY RESET
FOR SENIORS

**Balance Hormones, Reset Metabolism, and Lose Weight
with Delicious Recipes Designed to Get you in Shape**

D1528540

KHLOE FAULKNER

Contents

Introduction

Y ou've probably heard that once you hit 40, it's all downhill when it comes to your weight. That inexplicable force we call our metabolism does begin to grind a bit slower every year from age 30 onward. Well, that's true.

For some years now, diet and exercise trends have become only more extreme, as we've cut out larger and larger categories of foods and have exhausted ourselves at the gym. There was Paleo (no dairy, legumes, or grains), Whole 30 (same as Paleo, plus no alcohol), and keto (no carbs at all except for non-starchy vegetables), right on its heels. Now, intermittent fasting, by which you go sixteen hours a day or more without eating, or partial fasting, by which you eat only 500 calories a day one or more times a week, are the latest trends.

During this same period, extreme workouts came into vogue, and gyms specializing in high-intensity workouts sprouted across the nation. Yet our obsession with "healthy" eating and go-for-broke fitness hasn't left us any better off. It's just made eating an anxiety-producing activity.

To be honest, this obsession hasn't make us any healthier. According to Centers for Disease Control (CDC) 9.5 percent of Americans adults had diabetes in 2011, but this figure increased to 10.6 percent by the end of 2020. So, it's okay to think the only way to get healthy is to cut out huge chunks of different types of foods and knock yourself out at the gym.

1.

UNDERSTANDING WEIGHT LOSS WITH LIFESTYLE CHANGES

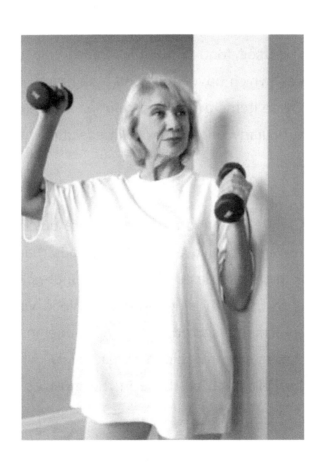

About Weight Loss with Lifestyle Changes

It's important to consider why we get overweight in the first place if you want to lose weight. The simple response, "because we consume so much and don't work out enough," is oversimplified. It's like talking to a tennis teacher and being advised that all you have to do to better your game is "take more scores than your competitor." True, but unsuccessful.

Why Do We Gain Weight as We Age?

So, why has there been such a global rise in obesity in the last 40 years? There are a variety of possible reasons, like elevated distress, fatigue, inadequate sleep, and a reduction in physical exercise, but more snacking and the reality that we are consuming a lot of processed food – not only more cola, cake, and sweets, but processed carbohydrates, which have increased by a massive 20% since 1980 – are at the top of the list. These items are rich in calories and very addicting. They mess with our hormones, particularly one hormone in specific: insulin since they're filled with sugar and refined fats.

Carbohydrates and insulin. Carbs, especially easily digestible carbs like those contained in fast food, white rice, and most bread, are quickly broken down in your stomach, releasing a torrent of glucose into your bloodstream. The effect is a burst of energy and a sugar 'high' that lasts just a few minutes. Sugar in the blood, on the other side, is toxic to the body since it affects blood vessels and nerves. As a result, the pancreas reacts by secreting the hormone insulin. Insulin's primary function is to rapidly lower elevated blood sugar levels, which it accomplishes by assisting energy-hungry cells such as those in the muscles and brain in absorbing the sugar.

However, if you eat regularly and do nothing to work off the calories, the body can grow more insulin resistant. As a consequence, the pancreas would function harder to generate rising levels of insulin. It's the equivalent of yelling at children. The louder you yell, the fewer they pay attention. Now two poor things happen:

1. When the body attempts to squeeze more and more calories onto your fat cells, they expand and get inflamed. You will reach your "personal fat threshold" at some stage. When there isn't enough room to comfortably store fat, it starts to expand into your vital organs, such as your liver. This is how the French prepare foie gras, or liver pâté. Geese are fed so much starchy grain that their livers quickly get bloated.

2. You're still starving, despite the fact that you're dragging so much weight around with you. Since you already have elevated insulin sensitivity, which promotes fat accumulation, this is the case. As a consequence, there is less food needed to sustain the majority of the body working. It's as though you're continually depositing cash into your savings account and still have a tough time removing it. You have it, but you can't seem to get your hands on it. Insulin resistance stops the body from obtaining and destroying its own accumulated energy. So, considering the fact that you have a lot of energy stored in the form of fat, your bodies and brain are unable to reach it.

3. Age has little effect on one's desire to lose weight. Research showed that weight control is not more challenging for older people, contrary to common opinion. Although several people believe that losing weight becomes more difficult when they become older, recent research finds that this is not the case. The results bring optimism to elderly people who continue to enjoy the health advantages of keeping a healthier weight.

Maintaining our wellbeing as we get older

"There is a range of explanations why people can ignore weight loss in the elderly," Dr. Barber notes. "These have an 'ageist' view that weight reduction is irrelevant to older people, as well as myths about older people's desire to shed weight by lifestyle changes and greater exercise." The research shows that weight management services conducted by medical practitioners, in fact, are beneficial. Dr. Barber recognizes that "older adults can believe that hospital-based obesity programs are not for them." "Service professionals and politicians should understand the value of weight reduction among older adults with obesity for the preservation of wellness and wellbeing, as well as the facilitation of safe aging," he writes. "Age does not lead in therapeutic judgments on the application of lifestyle management [in] older people," according to Dr. Barber.

Sleep, Stress and Weight Gain

We all feel guilty for gaining weight, and we believe it is solely our responsibility. After all, we've been advised countless times also that the main reason people gain weight is that they consume so much and don't get plenty of exercises. To put it another way, if we become big, it's because we're vain and lazy.

Fat gain isn't as easy as that, as we've already seen. Our minds and hormones can be hijacked by the foods we consume (absorbed and highly marketed by the food industry), whereas the environment we live in is designed to deter activity. Shopping malls are progressively located outside of town and can only be reached by vehicle. Cycling on roads is difficult, and although lifts are plentiful, stairs are not. We are often overwhelmed by temptation, which is difficult to avoid. The calorie-in, calorie-out crowd often overlooks the enormous value of tension. According to research, chronic stress has been linked to elevated appetite, comfort eating, self- loathing, and sleep disruption. This, in fact, adds to much more tension, as well as increased appetite, hunger, self-loathing, and so on.

You need a certain amount of tension in your life. It's important for life. When you're crossing the street and know you're going to be struck by a vehicle, the body can produce a surge of stress hormones, including adrenaline and cortisol, to brace you for actual movement.

The Importance of Physical Exercise

In common, many who survive to be a hundred years old in healthy living have been involved or rather active throughout their lives. Of these, there are variations. If you look at centenarians or maybe even your own immediate family, you're guaranteed to find somebody who defied the odds by consuming everything they liked, rarely walking, and yet living to a grand old age. According to Nir Barzilai of Albert Einstein College of Medicine, many Ashkenazi Jewish centenarians in New York are fully sedentary. Genetic factors are more certainly to blame for their long lives.

Genetic traits are obviously the most important element in deciding longevity. We know this because we've found mutants in mice and humans that have a strong level of defense towards age-related diseases. We all realize that even though a chimp follows a reasonable diet and exercises daily, he or she will never survive as long as a human. Sharing common 95% of our DNA chimps only live to be fifty years old. We have little influence on our biology. However, following dietary shifts, physical exercise is the second most important element in determining lifespan. The recommendations for exercise to improve fitness and lifespan are as follows:

Every day, go for a one-hour short walk. Running for an hour a day is a simple task to accomplish. Choose a cafe or restaurant fifteen minutes from your office and frequent it twice a day, for example. It can also be accomplished on weekends by cycling instead of driving.

Any second day, fly, drive or swim thirty to forty minutes, plus two hours on weekends. Using both a static and a road bike is the easiest way to accomplish this aim. If you can, cycle outside; if you can't, use a high-gear stationary bike (use a bike with high magnetic friction, which makes it difficult to wheel if you were riding up the hill). You could be sweating within ten minutes.

Since muscles only develop and retain or acquire strength in reaction to being challenged, any muscle in the body must be used regularly. Climbing six flights of stairs quickly, particularly if you haven't performed it in a number of years, may trigger leg pain. The stiffness is a symptom of a mild muscle injury. Muscle damage triggers the release of "muscle satellite cells" and, gradually, muscle development in the presence of enough proteins. Muscles may be partially damaged and healed when doing difficult routine activities. To stop both acute injury and the sluggish, permanent harm that comes with avoiding discomfort and continuing to exert weight on a damaged joint, muscle rehabilitation must be regulated.

2. BREAKFASTS

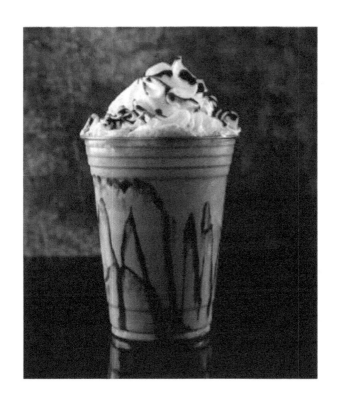

BREAKFAST GREEN SMOOTHIE

Prep Time: 5 minutes

Cook Time: 0 minutes

Total Time: 5 minutes

Yield: 1 serving

2 cups (60 g) spinach (or other leafy greens)

1/3 cup (46 g) raw almonds

2 Brazil nuts

1 cup (240 ml) coconut milk (unsweetened - from refrigerated cartons not cans)

1 scoop (20 g) greens powder (optional)

1 Tablespoon (10 g) psyllium seeds (or psyllium husks) or chia seeds

1. Place the spinach, almonds, Brazil nuts, and coconut milk into the blender first.
2. Blend until pureed.
3. Add in the rest of the ingredients (greens powder, psyllium seeds) and blend well.

Nutritional Data (estimates) - per serving:

Calories: 380 Fat: 30 g Net Carbohydrates: 5 g Protein: 12 g

BACON LEMON THYME MUFFINS

Prep Time: 10 minutes

Cook Time: 20 minutes

Total Time: 30 minutes

Yield: 12 servings

3 cups (360 g) almond flour

1 cup (100 g) bacon bits

1/2 cup (120 ml) ghee (or coconut oil), melted

4 eggs, whisked

2 teaspoons (2 g) lemon thyme (or use another herb of your choice)

1 teaspoon (4 g) baking soda

1/2 teaspoon (2 g) salt (optional)

1. Preheat oven to 350 F (175 C).
2. Melt the ghee in a mixing bowl.
3. Add in the rest of the ingredients except the bacon bits to the mixing bowl.
4. Mix everything together well.
5. Lastly, add in the bacon bits.
6. Line a muffin pan with muffin liners. Spoon the mixture into the muffin pan (to around 3/4 full).
7. Bake for 18-20 minutes until a toothpick comes out clean when you insert it into a muffin.

Nutritional Data (estimates) - per serving:

Calories: 300 Fat: 28 g Net Carbohydrates: 4 g Protein: 11 g

CREAMY BREAKFAST PORRIDGE

Prep Time: 2 minutes

Cook Time: 5 minutes

Total Time: 7 minutes

Yield: 2 servings

1/2 cup (60 g) almonds, ground using a food processor or blender

3/4 cup (180 ml) coconut milk

Erythritol or stevia to taste (optional)

1 teaspoon (2 g) cinnamon powder

Dash of nutmeg

Dash of cloves

Dash of cardamom (optional)

1. Heat the coconut milk in a small saucepan on medium heat until it forms a liquid.
2. Add in the ground almonds and sweetener and stir to mix in.
3. Keep stirring for approximately 5 minutes (it'll start to thicken a bit more).
4. Add in the spices (have a taste to check whether you want more sweetener or spices) and serve hot.

Nutritional Data (estimates) - per serving:

Calories: 430 Fat: 40 g Net Carbohydrates: 6 g Protein: 8 g

LEMON FRIED AVOCADOS

Prep Time: 2 minutes

Cook Time: 5 minutes

Total Time: 7 minutes

Yield: 2 servings

1 ripe avocado (not too soft), cut into slices

1 Tablespoon (15 ml) coconut oil

1 Tablespoon (15 ml) lemon juice

Salt to taste (or lemon salt)

1. Add coconut oil to a frying pan. Place the avocado slices into the oil gently.
2. Fry the avocado slices (turning gently) so that all sides are slightly browned.
3. Sprinkle the lemon juice and salt over the slices and serve warm

Nutritional Data (estimates) - per serving:

Calories: 200 Fat: 20 g Net Carbohydrates: 2 g Protein: 2 g

EASY SEED & NUT GRANOLA

Prep Time: 5 minutes

Cook Time: 0 minutes

Total Time: 5 minutes

Yield: 1 serving

Small handful of nuts (10 almonds, 3 Brazil nuts, 5 cashews)

2 Tablespoons (17 g) pumpkin seeds

1 Tablespoon (12 g) cacao nibs

1 Tablespoon (5 g) coconut flakes

1/4 cup (60 ml) unsweetened coconut or almond milk

1. Mix together all the dry ingredients. If you're making a large batch, then store leftovers in an airtight container. Serve with coconut or almond milk.

Nutritional Data (estimates) - per serving:

Calories: 400 Fat: 30 g Net Carbohydrates: 9 g Protein: 9 g

ALMOND BUTTER CHOCO SHAKE

Prep Time: 5 minutes

Cook Time: 0 minutes

Total Time: 5 minutes

Yield: 1 serving

1 cup (240 ml) coconut milk or almond milk

2 Tablespoons (10 g) unsweetened cacao powder (or 1 scoop CoBionic Indulgence for added collagen)

1 Tablespoon (16 g) almond butter

1 teaspoon (5 ml) vanilla extract

1/4 cup (35 g) ice (optional)

Erythritol or stevia to taste (optional)

1. Place all the ingredients into a blender and blend well.

Nutritional Data (estimates) - per serving:

Calories: 190 Fat: 15 g Net Carbohydrates: 7 g Protein: 4 g

EGG AND HAM ROLLS

Prep Time: 10 minutes

Cook Time: 15 minutes

Total Time: 25 minutes

Yield: 4 servings

4 slices of ham

1 cucumber, sliced thin

4 eggs, whisked well

2 Tablespoons (30 ml) avocado oil, to cook with

1. Add 1 teaspoon of avocado oil to a frying pan on low to medium heat and spread it around with a paper towel.
2. Add 1/4 cup of whisked eggs to the pan and roll it around to spread it thin.
3. Place a lid on top of the frying pan and let it cook until the base of the egg wrap is cooked (approx. 2-3 minutes). Carefully place on a plate and let cool.
4. Repeat in batches with the rest of the egg mixture to make egg wraps.
5. Create rolls with the egg wraps, slices of ham, and cucumber slices.

Nutritional Data (estimates) - per serving:

Calories: 158 Fat: 12 g Net Carbohydrates: 1 g Protein: 12 g

KALE AND CHIVES EGG MUFFINS

Prep Time: 10 minutes

Cook Time: 30 minutes

Total Time: 40 minutes

Yield: 4 servings

6 eggs

1 cup kale, finely chopped

1/4 cup (17 g) chives, finely chopped

1/2 cup (120 ml) almond or coconut milk

Salt and pepper to taste

8 slices of prosciutto or bacon (optional)

1. Preheat the oven to 350 F (175 C).
2. Whisk the eggs and add in the chopped kale and chives. Also add in the almond/coconut milk, salt, and pepper. Mix well.
3. Grease 8 muffin cups with coconut oil or line each cup with a prosciutto slice.
4. Divide the egg mixture between the 8 muffin cups. Fill only 2/3 of each cup as the mixture rises when it's baking.
5. Bake in oven for 30 minutes.
6. Let cool a few minutes and then lift out carefully with a fork. Note that the muffins will sink a bit.

Nutritional Data (estimates) - per serving:

Calories: 240 Fat: 20 g Net Carbohydrates: 3 g Protein: 12 g

BREAKFAST TURKEY WRAP

Prep Time: 5 minutes

Cook Time: 20 minutes

Total Time: 25 minutes

Yield: 1 serving

2 slices of turkey breast (use more if the slices break easily)

2 romaine lettuce leaves (or 2 slices of avocado)

2 slices of bacon

1 Tablespoon (15 ml) coconut oil to cook in

1. Cook the 2 slices of bacon to the crispness you like.
2. Scramble the 2 eggs in the coconut oil (or bacon fat).
3. Make 2 wraps by placing half the scrambled eggs, 1 slice of bacon, and 1 romaine lettuce leaf on each slice of turkey breast.

Nutritional Data (estimates) - per serving:

Calories: 360 Fat: 30 g Net Carbohydrates: 3 g Protein: 20 g

EASY BACON CUPS

Prep Time: 15 minutes

Cook Time: 25 minutes

Total Time: 40 minutes

Yield: 4 servings

20 thin slices of bacon

Equipment: standard nonstick metal muffin or cupcake pan

1. Preheat oven to 400 F (200 C).
2. Each bacon cup will require 2 and 1/2 slices of bacon.
3. Start by turning the entire muffin/cupcake pan over, so that the side that is normally the bottom is on top. To make 1 bacon cup, place 2 half slices of bacon across the back of one of the muffin/cupcake cups, both in the same direction. Then, place another half slice across those 2, perpendicular to the direction of the first 2 half slices. Finally, wrap a whole slice of bacon tightly around the sides of the cup. The slice wrapped around the sides will help to hold the bottom pieces of bacon together.
4. Repeat Step #3 for the other cups.
5. Place the entire pan (still upside-down) into the oven and bake for 25 minutes until crispy (place a baking tray underneath in the oven to catch any dripping bacon fat).

Nutritional Data (estimates) - per serving:

Calories: 180 Fat: 18 g Net Carbohydrates: 0 g Protein: 5 g

3. APPETIZERS

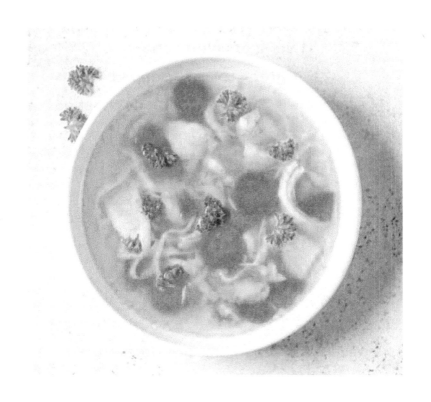

CHICKEN NOODLE SOUP

Prep Time: 15 minutes

Cook Time: 15 minutes

Total Time: 30 minutes

Yield: 2 servings

3 cups (720 ml) chicken broth or bone broth

1 chicken breast (approx 225 g or 0.5 lb), chopped into small pieces

2 Tablespoons (30 ml) avocado oil

1 stalk of celery, chopped

1 green onion, chopped

1/4 cup (8 g) cilantro, finely chopped

1 zucchini, peeled

Salt to taste

1. Add the avocado oil into a saucepan and saute the diced chicken in there until cooked.
2. Add chicken broth to the same saucepan and simmer.
3. Add the chopped celery and green onion into the saucepan.
4. Create zucchini noodles – I used a potato peeler to create long strands, but other options include using a spiralizer or a food processor with the shredding attachment.
5. Add zucchini noodles and finely chopped cilantro to the saucepan. Simmer for a few more minutes, add salt to taste, and serve immediately.

Nutritional Data (estimates) - per serving:

Calories: 310 Fat: 16 g Net Carbohydrates: 4 g Protein: 34 g

BACON WRAPPED CHICKEN BITES WITH GARLIC MAYO

Prep Time: 10 minutes

Cook Time: 30 minutes

Total Time: 40 minutes

Yield: 4 servings

1 large chicken breast (approx 225 g or 0.5 lb), cut into small bites (approx. 22-27 pieces)

8-9 thin slices of bacon, cut into thirds

3 Tablespoons (30 g) garlic powder

For the garlic mayo:

1/4 cup (60 ml) mayo (see page 125 for recipe)

2 cloves of garlic, minced

Dash of salt

Dash of chili powder (optional)

1 teaspoon (5 ml) lemon juice (optional)

1 teaspoon (4 g) garlic powder (optional)

1. Preheat oven to 400 F (200 C) and line a baking tray with foil.
2. Place the garlic power into a small bowl and dip each small chunk of chicken in it.
3. Wrap each short bacon piece around each garlic powder-dipped piece of chicken. Place the bacon wrapped chicken bites on the baking tray. (Try to space them out so they're not touching on the tray.)
4. Bake for 25-30 minutes until the bacon turns crispy.
5. Meanwhile, combine the garlic mayo ingredients in a small bowl and use a fork to whisk it slightly.
6. Serve the bacon wrapped chicken bites with cocktail sticks and the garlic mayo.

Nutritional Data (estimates) - per serving:

Calories: 280 Fat: 25 g Net Carbohydrates: 7 g Protein: 7 g

FIERY BUFFALO WINGS

Prep Time: 15 minutes

Cook Time: 45 minutes

Total Time: 1 hour

Yield: 4 servings

12 small chicken wings

1/2 cup (56 g) coconut flour

1/2 teaspoon (1 g) cayenne pepper

1/2 teaspoon (1 g) black pepper

1/2 teaspoon (1 g) crushed red pepper flakes

1 Tablespoon (7 g) paprika

1 Tablespoon (8 g) garlic powder

1 Tablespoon (15 g) salt

1/4 cup (60 ml) ghee, melted

1/4 cup (60 ml) hot sauce

1. Preheat oven to 400 F (200 C).
2. Mix the coconut flour, dried spices, and salt together in a bowl.
3. Coat each chicken wing with the coconut flour mixture. Refrigerate for 15-30 minutes to help the flour stick a bit better to the wings (optional).
4. Grease a baking tray (or line it with aluminum foil).
5. Mix the ghee and the hot sauce together well.
6. Dip each chicken wing into the ghee and hot sauce mixture and place onto the baking tray.
7. Bake for 45 minutes.

Nutritional Data (estimates) - per serving:

Calories: 500 Fat: 38 g Net Carbohydrates: 3 g Protein: 29

EASY EGG DROP SOUP

Prep Time: 5 minutes

Cook Time: 10 minutes

Total Time: 15 minutes

Yield: 1 serving

2 cups (480 ml) chicken broth or bone broth

1/4 cup (17 g) scallions (chopped green onions)

1/2 tomato, sliced

1 egg, whisked

1 Tablespoon (15 ml) tamari sauce

1/2 teaspoon (1 g) fresh ginger, grated (optional)

Salt and pepper to taste

1. Heat up the chicken broth (or other broth) in a saucepan.

2. Slowly drizzle in whisked egg and stir slowly clockwise until ribbons form.

3. Add in rest of ingredients and let it cook for a few minutes.

Nutritional Data (estimates) - per serving:

Calories: 130 Fat: 5 g Net Carbohydrates: 5 g Protein: 15 g

CRAB HASH WITH GINGER AND CILANTRO

Prep Time: 10 minutes

Cook Time: 15 minutes

Total Time: 25 minutes

Yield: 4-6 servings

2 zucchinis, peeled and shredded

1 lb (454 g) lump crabmeat (fresh or canned)

1/4 cup (17 g) scallions (green onions) chopped (optional)

1/4 cup (8 g) cilantro, finely chopped

2 cloves of garlic, minced

2 teaspoons (4 g) fresh ginger, grated

1 Tablespoon (15 ml) lemon juice

2 boiled eggs, diced (optional)

Salt to taste

2 Tablespoons (30 ml) coconut oil

1. Place 2 Tablespoons of coconut oil into a frying pan (or a saucepan).
2. Add in the shredded zucchinis, crabmeat, and scallions and sauté for 5-10 minutes.
3. Lastly, add the cilantro, garlic, ginger, lemon juice, and salt to taste. Sauté for a few minutes more to combine the flavors.
4. Top with the diced boiled eggs (optional) and serve immediately.

SUBSTITUTIONS

• Chicken breast (finely diced) can be used instead of crabmeat, but you should cook it separately first.

• Scrambled eggs can be used instead of boiled eggs.

• Apple cider vinegar can be used instead of lemon juice.

Nutritional Data (estimates) - per serving:

Calories: 150 Fat: 7 g Net Carbohydrates: 2 g Protein: 19 g

BIG EASY SALAD

Prep Time: 15 minutes

Cook Time: 0 minutes

Total Time: 15 minutes

Yield: 2 servings

2 romaine lettuce, chopped into small pieces

10 cherry or grape tomatoes

1 Tablespoon (4 g) sliced almonds (optional)

4-6 slices of bacon, cooked (crumbled)

1/2 lb (225 g) ham, diced

Olive oil and lemon juice as dressing

1. Add all the ingredients together and toss with olive oil and small amount of lemon juice to taste.

Nutritional Data (estimates) - per serving:

Calories: 570 Fat: 36 g Net Carbohydrates: 10 g Protein: 40 g

ASIAN DEVILED EGGS

Prep Time: 10 minutes

Cook Time: 10 minutes

Total Time: 20 minutes

Yield: 16 servings

16 eggs

1 Tablespoon (15 ml) sesame oil

3 Tablespoons (45 ml) avocado oil

3 Tablespoons (45 ml) tamari sauce

1 teaspoon (5 ml) mustard

2 Tablespoons chives, finely diced

1 red chili pepper, finely sliced

1. Soft boil the eggs.
2. Slice each egg in half lengthwise.
3. Remove the yolks and set aside in a bowl. Mash or blend the yolks with the sesame oil, avocado oil, tamari sauce, and mustard.
4. Place the yolk mixture back into the egg whites (use piping bags or a small spoon).
5. Sprinkle the chives on top of the egg halves and place one slice of red chili pepper on top of each deviled egg half.

Nutritional Data (estimates) - per serving:

Calories: 93 Fat: 8 g Net Carbohydrates: 0 g Protein: 6 g

RED CABBAGE SOUP

Prep Time: 15 minutes

Cook Time: 25 minutes

Total Time: 40 minutes

Yield: 8 servings

1 red cabbage, sliced

1/4 onion, chopped

4 stalks of celery, chopped

1 bell pepper, chopped

8 cups (2 l) chicken broth or bone broth

2 tomatoes, chopped

3 Tablespoons (45 ml) avocado oil, to cook with

1/4 cup bacon bits (optional)

Salt and pepper, to taste

1. Add avocado oil to a large pot and then saute the cabbage, onions, celery, and bell pepper for 3 minutes on high heat.
2. Pour in the broth and add in the chopped tomatoes.
3. Bring to a boil and then simmer for 20 minutes until the cabbage is tender. Season with salt and pepper, to taste, and top with some bacon bits (optional).

Nutritional Data (estimates) - per serving:

Calories: 128 Fat: 10 g Net Carbohydrates: 4 g Protein: 2 g

4. FISH AND SEAFOOD

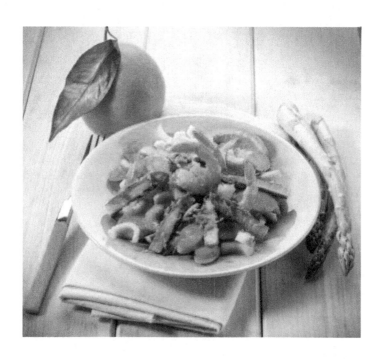

BREADED COD WITH GARLIC GHEE SAUCE

Prep Time: 10 minutes

Cook Time: 20 minutes

Total Time: 30 minutes

Yield: 4 servings

4 cod filets (approx. 0.3 lb or 136 g each)

1/2 cup (30 g) coconut flour (or almond flour)

2 Tablespoons (15 g) coconut flakes

3 Tablespoons (30 g) garlic powder

1 Tablespoon (7 g) onion powder

1 egg, whisked

Salt to taste

2 Tablespoons (30 ml) ghee

3 cloves of garlic, minced

Coconut oil for greasing baking tray

1. Preheat oven to 425 F (220 C).
2. In a large bowl, whisk an egg.
3. In a separate large bowl, combine the breading ingredients (coconut flour, coconut flakes, garlic powder, and onion powder). Add in salt and taste the mixture to see how much salt you like.
4. Cover a baking tray with aluminum foil and grease with coconut oil.
5. Dip each cod filet first into the whisked egg and then into the breading mixture and cover it well with the breading. Place the breaded cod onto the baking tray.
6. Bake for 15-20 minutes until the cod flakes easily.
7. While the cod is in the oven, prepare the garlic ghee sauce by melting the ghee slightly and adding in the minced garlic.
8. Pour the garlic ghee sauce on top of the breaded cod and serve.

Nutritional Data (estimates) - per serving:
Calories: 280 Fat: 15 g Net Carbohydrates: 5 g Protein: 25 g

FISH TACOS

Prep Time: 30 minutes

Cook Time: 15 minutes

Total Time: 45 minutes

Yield: 2 servings

For the fish:

1 lb (454 g) tilapia (halibut/cod), cut into 1/2 inch by 3/4 inch (1 cm by 2 cm) strips

1/2 cup (56 g) coconut flour

1 Tablespoon (10 g) garlic powder

2 teaspoons (10 g) salt

2 teaspoons (5 g) cumin powder

Coconut oil for frying

For the white sauce:

1/2 cup (120 g) mayo (see page 125)

1 Tablespoon (15 ml) lime juice

1 teaspoon (2 g) dried oregano

1/2 teaspoon (1 g) cumin powder

Dash of chili powder

To eat:

4-6 lettuce leaves

1/4 cup (60 g) salsa (optional)

2 Tablespoons (4 g) cilantro, chopped

4-6 lime wedges

1. To make the white sauce, mix all the sauce ingredients together with a fork.
2. Mix together the coconut flour, garlic powder, cumin powder, and salt in a bowl.
3. Drop the fish strips into the bowl and coat with the coconut flour mixture.
4. Heat up coconut oil in a saucepan on high heat (the coconut oil should be approx. 1/2 inch (1-2 cm) deep).
5. Carefully add the coated fish strips to the hot coconut oil.

6. Fry until the coconut flour coating turns a golden brown color (approx. 5 minutes).
7. Place fried fish strips in a bowl lined with a paper towel to soak up excess oil.
8. To eat, place fish strips on a lettuce leaf with salsa, cilantro, and white sauce. Serve with lime wedges.

Nutritional Data (estimates) - per serving:

Calories: 400 Fat: 15 g Net Carbohydrates: 9 g Protein: 50 g

POPCORN SHRIMP

Prep Time: 5 minutes

Cook Time: 20 minutes

Total Time: 25 minutes

Yield: 2 servings

1/2 lb (225 g) small shrimp, peeled

2 eggs, whisked

6 Tablespoons (36 g) cajun seasoning

6 Tablespoons (42 g) coconut flour

Coconut oil for frying

1. Melt the coconut oil in a saucepan (use enough coconut oil so that it's ½ inch (1-2 cm) deep) or deep fryer.
2. Place the whisked eggs into a large bowl, and in another large bowl, combine the coconut flour and seasoning.
3. Drop a handful of the shrimp into the whisked eggs and stir around so that each shrimp is coated.
4. Then take the shrimp out of the whisked eggs and place into the seasoning bowl. Coat the shrimp with the coconut flour and seasoning mixture.
5. Place the coated shrimp into the hot oil and fry until golden. Try not to stir the pot and don't place too many shrimp into the pot at once (make sure all the shrimp is touching the oil).

6. Using a slotted spoon, remove the shrimp and place on paper towels to absorb the excess oil. Repeat for the rest of the shrimp (change the oil if there are too many solids in it).

7. Cool for 10 minutes (the outside will get crisp).

Nutritional Data (estimates) - per serving:

Calories: 390 Fat: 23 g Net Carbohydrates: 3 g Protein: 30 g

ROSEMARY BAKED SALMON

Prep Time: 5 minutes

Cook Time: 30 minutes

Total Time: 35 minutes

Yield: 2 servings

2 salmon filets (fresh or defrosted)

1 Tablespoon (2 g) fresh rosemary leaves

1/4 cup (60 ml) olive oil

1 teaspoon (5 g) salt (optional or to taste)

1. Preheat oven to 350 F (175 C).

2. Mix the olive oil, rosemary, and salt together in a bowl.

3. Place one salmon filet at a time into the mixture and rub mixture onto the filet.

4. Wrap each filet in a piece of aluminum foil with some of the remaining mixture.

5. Bake for 25-30 minutes.

Nutritional Data (estimates) - per serving:

Calories: 430 Fat: 18 g Net Carbohydrates: 0 g Protein: 63 g

EASY SALMON STEW

Prep Time: 10 minutes

Cook Time: 20 minutes

Total Time: 30 minutes

Yield: 2 servings

4 cups (1 l) chicken broth (or bone broth)

2 salmon filets (1/2 lb or 225 g), diced

2 zucchinis, diced

4 button mushrooms, diced

2 cups (200 g) chopped celery

1/2 cup (16 g) chopped cilantro

Salt and pepper (to taste)

1. Place all the vegetables with the broth into a pot and simmer for 15 minutes.

2. Add the diced salmon and simmer for another 5 minutes. Add salt and pepper.

Nutritional Data (estimates) - per serving:

Calories: 450 Fat: 12 g Net Carbohydrates: 7 g Protein: 70 g

CUCUMBER GINGER SHRIMP

Prep Time: 5 minutes

Cook Time: 10 minutes

Total Time: 15 minutes

Yield: 1 serving

1 large cucumber, peeled and sliced into 1/2-inch round slices

10-15 large shrimp/prawns (defrosted if frozen)

1 teaspoon (1 g) fresh ginger, grated

Salt to taste

Coconut oil to cook with

1. Place 1 Tablespoon (15 ml) of coconut oil into a frying pan on medium heat.

2. Add in the ginger and the cucumber and sauté for 2-3 minutes.

3. Add in the shrimp and cook until they turn pink and are no longer translucent.

4. Add salt to taste and serve.

Nutritional Data (estimates) - per serving:

Calories: 250 Fat: 16 g Net Carbohydrates: 4 g Protein: 20 g

AVOCADO TUNA BOWL WITH TAHINI TAMARI PASTE

Prep Time: 10 minutes

Cook Time: 0 minutes

Total Time: 10 minutes

Yield: 2 servings

1 large avocado, destoned and diced

2 Tablespoons (30 ml) lime juice

2 Tablespoons (30 ml) olive oil, to cook with

2 cans of tuna (340 g or 12 oz), drained and flaked

2 Tablespoons of fresh cilantro, finely chopped

2 Tablespoons (30 ml) tahini sauce

3 Tablespoons (45 ml) gluten-free tamari sauce or coconut aminos

1 Tablespoon (15 ml) sesame oil

1. To make the tahini tamari paste, mix together the tahini, tamari sauce, and sesame oil.
2. To make the tuna salad, mix the lime juice, cilantro, olive oil, and tuna together.
3. To serve, place the diced avocado into a bowl, then top with the tuna and paste.

Nutritional Data (estimates) - per serving:

Calories: 667 Fat: 48 g Net Carbohydrates: 7 g Protein: 46 g

5. CHICKEN ENTREES

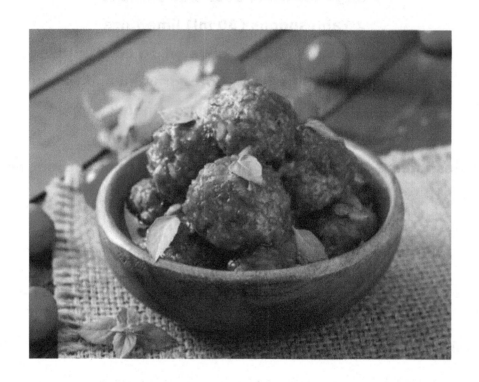

GRILLED CHICKEN SKEWERS WITH GARLIC SAUCE

Prep Time: 15 minutes

Cook Time: 15 minutes

Total Time: 30 minutes

Yield: 2 servings

For the skewers:

1 lb (454 g) chicken breast, cut into large cubes (approx 1-inch)

1 onion, chopped

2 bell peppers, chopped

1 zucchini

For the garlic sauce:

1 head of garlic, peeled

1 teaspoon (5 g) salt

Approx. 1/4 cup (60 ml) lemon juice

Approx. 1 cup (240 ml) olive oil

For the marinade:

1/2 cup (120 ml) olive oil

1 teaspoon (5 g) salt

1. Heat up the grill to high. If using wooden skewers, soak them in water first.
2. For the garlic sauce, place the garlic cloves and salt into the blender. Then add in around 1/8 cup of the lemon juice and 1/2 cup of olive oil.
3. Blend well for 5-10 seconds, then slow your blender down and drizzle in more lemon juice and olive oil alternatively until it forms a smooth consistency.
4. Keep half the garlic sauce to serve with.
5. Take the other half of the garlic sauce and add in the additional 1/2 cup of olive oil and teaspoon of salt. Mix well - this makes the marinade.
6. Chop the chicken, onion, bell peppers, and zucchini into approximate 1-inch cubes or squares. Mix them in a bowl with the marinade.

7. Place the cubes on skewers and grill on high until the chicken is cooked (usually, we grill on the bottom for a few minutes to get the charred look and then move the skewers to a top rack with the lid down to cook the chicken well).
8. Serve with the garlic sauce you kept.

Nutritional Data (estimates) - per serving:

Calories: 580 Fat: 33 g Net Carbohydrates: 9 g Protein: 55 g

SPINACH BASIL CHICKEN MEATBALLS

Prep Time: 10 minutes

Cook Time: 15 minutes

Total Time: 25 minutes

Yield: 2 servings

2 chicken breasts (approx. 1 lb or 454 g)

1/4 lb (115 g) spinach

2 teaspoons (10 g) salt

10 basil leaves

5 cloves of garlic, peeled

3 Tablespoons (45 ml) olive oil

2 Tablespoons (30 ml) olive oil or avocado oil to cook in

1. Place the chicken breasts, spinach, salt, basil leaves, garlic, and 3 Tablespoons of olive oil into a food processor and process well.
2. Make ping-pong ball sized meatballs from the meat mixture.
3. Add the 2 Tablespoons olive oil or avocado oil to a frying pan and fry the meatballs for 4 minutes on medium heat (fry in 2 batches if necessary). Turn the meatballs and fry for another 10 minutes. Make sure the meatballs don't get burnt.
4. Check the meatballs are fully cooked by cutting into one or using a meat thermometer.

Nutritional Data (estimates) - per serving:

Calories: 600 Fat: 40 g Net Carbohydrates: 4 g Protein: 55 g

THAI CHICKEN AND RICE

Prep Time: 10 minutes

Cook Time: 15 minutes

Total Time: 25 minutes

Yield: 4 servings

1 head of cauliflower

Meat from a small roasted chicken (or use 3 cooked chicken breasts), shredded (or use some leftover meat)

2 eggs, whisked

1 Tablespoon (5 g) fresh ginger, grated

3 cloves of garlic, minced

1 Tablespoon (15 ml) tamari sauce

1/2 cup (16 g) cilantro, chopped

4 Tablespoons (60 ml) coconut oil to cook with

Salt and pepper to taste

1. If you don't have cooked shredded chicken, poach 3 chicken breasts and shred them or use another leftover meat.
2. Break the cauliflower into florets and food process until it forms a rice-like texture (may need to be done in batches). Squeeze excess water out.
3. Scramble 2 eggs in some coconut oil. Lightly salt the scrambled eggs and put aside while you make the cauliflower rice.
4. Place the cauliflower "rice" into a large pan with coconut oil and cook the cauliflower rice (may need to be done in 2 pans or in batches). Keep the heat on medium and stir regularly for 10 minutes.
5. Add in the shredded chicken, scrambled eggs, ginger, garlic, tamari sauce, cilantro, salt, and pepper to taste. Mix together, cook for another 2-3 minutes and serve.

Nutritional Data (estimates) - per serving:

Calories: 480 Fat: 31 g Net Carbohydrates: 4 g Protein: 41 g

PAN-FRIED ITALIAN CHICKEN TENDERS

Prep Time: 15 minutes

Cook Time: 15 minutes

Total Time: 30 minutes

Yield: 2 servings

1 lb (454 g) chicken tenders (approx. 12 chicken tenders)

2/3 cup (160 ml) olive oil + more for cooking

2 Tablespoons (30 ml) lime juice or white wine vinegar

1.5 Tablespoons (20 g) mustard

2 teaspoons (2 g) Italian seasoning

4 cloves of garlic

1 teaspoon (5 g) salt and to taste

Salad leaves

1. Place the olive oil, lime juice or vinegar, mustard, Italian seasoning, garlic, and 1 teaspoon salt into the blender and blend well.
2. Heat up a frying pan and place 2 Tablespoons of olive oil into it. Place half the chicken tenders into the pan and cook on medium to high heat. Add in 1/3 of the mixture from the blender into the frying pan, coating the chicken tenders.
3. After 3-4 minutes, flip the chicken tenders (they should be browned) and cook the other side for 2-3 minutes until done. Test using a meat thermometer or cut one open to see if the chicken is cooked through. Repeat for the rest of the chicken tenders (if you have 2 frying pans, you can cook both batches simultaneously).
4. Divide the salad between 2 plates and place 6 cooked chicken tenders on top of each salad. Serve with the rest of the sauce from the blender.

Nutritional Data (estimates) - per serving:

Calories: 600 Fat: 35 g Net Carbohydrates: 3 g Protein: 55 g

CHICKEN NUGGETS

Prep Time: 10 minutes

Cook Time: 15 minutes

Total Time: 25 minutes

Yield: 2 servings

2 chicken breasts, cut into cubes

1/2 cup (56 g) coconut flour

1 egg

2 Tablespoons (20 g) garlic powder

1 teaspoon (5 g) salt (or to taste)

1/4-1/2 cup (60-120 ml) ghee for shallow frying

1. Cube the chicken breasts if you haven't done so already.
2. In a bowl, mix together the coconut flour, garlic powder, and salt. Taste the mixture to see if you'd like more salt.
3. In a separate bowl, whisk 1 egg to make the egg wash.
4. Place the ghee in a saucepan on medium heat (or use a deep fryer).
5. Dip the cubed chicken in the egg wash and then drop into the coconut flour mixture to coat it with the "breading."
6. Carefully place some of the "breaded" chicken cubes into the ghee and fry until golden (approx. 10 minutes). Make sure there's only a single layer of chicken in the pan so that they can all cook in the oil. Turn the chicken pieces to make sure they get cooked uniformly. Depending on the size of the pan, you might need to do this step in batches.
7. Place the cooked chicken pieces onto paper towels to soak up any excess oil. Enjoy by themselves or with some coconut ranch dressing or garlic sauce.

Nutritional Data (estimates) - per serving:

Calories: 550 Fat: 27 g Net Carbohydrates: 8 g Protein: 60 g

COCONUT CHICKEN CURRY

Prep Time: 15 minutes

Cook Time: 50 minutes

Total Time: 1 hour 5 minutes

Yield: 4 servings

3 chicken breasts, cut into chunks

1 Tablespoon (15 ml) ghee or coconut oil

1 cup (240 ml) coconut cream (the top layer of cream from a refrigerated can of coconut milk)

1 cup (240 ml) chicken broth

2 cups (250 g) carrots (or zucchini), diced

1 cup (100 g) celery, chopped

2 tomatoes, diced

1 Tablespoon (5 g) fresh ginger, grated

1.5 Tablespoons (10 g) curry powder or garam masala

1/4 cup (8 g) cilantro, roughly chopped

6 cloves of garlic, minced

Salt to taste

1. Sauté the chicken in the ghee in a medium-sized saucepan.
2. When the outside of the chicken has all turned white, add in the coconut cream and the chicken broth and mix well.
3. Add in the carrots, celery, and tomatoes.
4. Add in the ginger and curry powder (or garam masala).
5. Cook on medium heat with the lid on for 40 minutes (stirring occasionally).
6. Add in the cilantro, minced garlic, and salt to taste. Cook for another 5 minutes and serve. Enjoy by itself, with a slice of Microwave Quick Bread, or with some Cauliflower White "Rice".

Nutritional Data (estimates) - per serving:

Calories: 450 Fat: 25 g Net Carbohydrates: 9 g Protein: 45 g

PRESSURE COOKER CHICKEN STEW

Prep Time: 15 minutes

Cook Time: 35 minutes

Total Time: 50 minutes

Yield: 3 servings

2-3 chicken breasts (approx. 1 lb or 454 g), diced

4 cups (1 l) chicken broth or bone broth

2 small carrots, chopped

3 stalks of celery, chopped

1/2 onion, chopped

1 teaspoon (5 ml) tamari sauce

1/2 Tablespoon (1 g) fresh thyme leaves (or use 1/2 tsp (0.5 g) dried thyme)

1/2 cup (15 g) parsley, chopped and divided (save half for when you're serving)

1 Tablespoon (7 g) unflavored gelatin powder (optional)

Salt to taste

1. Place the diced chicken breasts, chicken broth, chopped carrots, chopped celery, chopped onion, tamari sauce, thyme, and half the parsley into the pressure cooker pot.
2. If you're adding in gelatin, then stir it in until it dissolves.
3. Set the pressure cooker on high pressure for 35 minutes. When ready, follow your pressure cooker's instructions for releasing the pressure safely.
4. Add salt to taste and sprinkle in the rest of the chopped parsley.

Nutritional Data (estimates) - per serving:

Calories: 250 Fat: 4 g Net Carbohydrates: 4 g Protein: 44 g

CHICKEN BACON BURGERS

Prep Time: 10 minutes

Cook Time: 15 minutes

Total Time: 25 minutes

Yield: 8 servings

4 chicken breasts

4 slices of bacon

1/4 medium onion

2 cloves of garlic

1/4 cup (60 ml) avocado oil, to cook with

1. Food process the chicken, bacon, onion and garlic and form 8 patties. You might need to do this in batches.
2. Fry patties in the avocado oil in batches. Make sure burgers are fully cooked.
3. Serve with guacamole.

Nutritional Data (estimates) - per serving:

Calories: 319 Fat: 24 g Net Carbohydrates: 1 g Protein: 25 g

BASIL CHICKEN SAUTE

Prep Time: 10 minutes

Cook Time: 15 minutes

Total Time: 25 minutes

Yield: 2 servings

1 chicken breast (0.5 lb or 225 g), minced or chopped very small

2 cloves of garlic, minced

1 chili pepper, diced (optional)

1 cup (1 large bunch) basil leaves, finely chopped

1 Tablespoon (15 ml) tamari sauce

2 Tablespoons (30 ml) avocado or coconut oil to cook in

Salt, to taste

1. Add oil to a frying pan and saute the garlic and pepper.
2. Then add in the minced chicken and saute until the chicken is cooked.
3. Add the tamari sauce and salt to taste. Add in the basil leaves and mix it in.

Nutritional Data (estimates) - per serving:

Calories: 320 Fat: 24 g Net Carbohydrates: 2 g Protein: 24 g

6. BEEF & PORK ENTREES

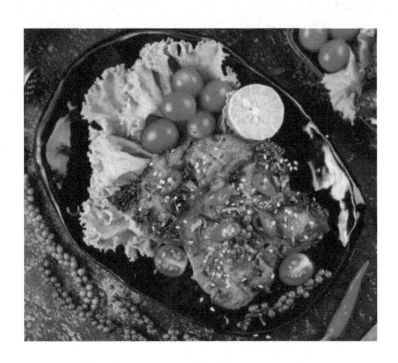

ZUCCHINI BEEF PHO

Prep Time: 15 minutes

Cook Time: 10 minutes

Total Time: 25 minutes

Yield: 2 servings

3 cups (720 ml) chicken/beef broth or bone broth

1/2 lb (225 g) beef round, sliced very thin

1 teaspoon (1 g) fresh ginger, grated (or use 1/2 teaspoon (1 g) ginger powder)

1/2 teaspoon (1 g) cinnamon powder

2 green onions, diced (scallions)

1/4 cup (8 g) cilantro, finely diced

2 zucchinis, shredded (or 2 packs of shirataki noodles)

Salt and pepper to taste

10 basil leaves

1/2 lime, cut into 4 wedges

1. Slice the beef round very thinly against the grain (tip: freeze the beef for 20- 30 minutes before slicing to get thinner slices).
2. Heat up the broth.
3. When the broth starts boiling, add in the freshly grated ginger, cinnamon powder, and salt and pepper to taste.
4. Add in the beef slices slowly, making sure they don't all clump together.
5. Then add in the zucchini noodles, the green onions, and the cilantro.
6. Cook for 1 minute until the beef slices are done.
7. Serve with the basil leaves and lime wedges.

Nutritional Data (estimates) - per serving:

Calories: 300 Fat: 14 g Net Carbohydrates: 7 g Protein: 30 g

MEXICAN TACOS

Prep Time: 15 minutes

Cook Time: 15 minutes

Total Time: 30 minutes

Yield: 2 servings

1 lb (454 g) ground beef

1 small onion, diced

2 tomatoes, diced

1 bell pepper, diced

1 jalapeño pepper, deseeded and diced

2 cloves of garlic, minced

1 Tablespoon (6 g) cumin powder

1 Tablespoon (6 g) paprika

1 Tablespoon (5 g) dried oregano

1/4 teaspoon (0.5 g) chili powder (or to taste)

Salt and pepper to taste

1/4 cup (8 g) cilantro, finely chopped (for garnish)

1 Tablespoon (15 ml) coconut oil to cook with

Lettuce leaves to serve with

1. Sauté the onions in the coconut oil until the onions turn translucent.
2. Add in the ground beef and sauté until the beef is pretty much cooked (turns light brown). Use a spatula to stir the beef to ensure it doesn't clump together. Pour out any excess water/oil produced during cooking.
3. When the beef is pretty much cooked, add in the tomatoes, bell pepper, jalapeño pepper, minced garlic, cumin powder, paprika, oregano, chili powder, salt, and pepper.
4. Cook until the tomatoes and peppers are soft.
5. Garnish with cilantro and serve with lettuce wraps or by themselves.

Nutritional Data (estimates) - per serving:

Calories: 560 Fat: 37 g Net Carbohydrates: 7 g Protein: 47 g

MINI BURGERS

Prep Time: 10 minutes

Cook Time: 20 minutes

Total Time: 30 minutes

Yield: 4 servings

12 oz (340 g) ground beef

2 Tablespoons (28 g) mustard

Pickles (optional)

A few lettuce leaves

Salt to taste

2 Tablespoons (30 ml) avocado oil (or coconut oil or ghee), to cook with

For "burger buns:"

2/3 cup (70 g) almond flour

1 teaspoon (4 g) baking powder

1 teaspoon (5 g) salt

2 eggs

5 Tablespoons (75 ml) avocado oil (or coconut oil or ghee), melted

1. Make 4 small thin patties with the ground beef (each should be approx. 2-inch across in diameter).
2. Place avocado oil into a frying pan and fry the burger patties on medium to high heat. Fry for 2 minutes on each side until both sides are well browned (this is around medium in terms of rareness for the patties).
3. After the patties are cooked, salt them lightly and place them on a plate to drain.
4. Meanwhile, take 2 mugs and divide the burger bun ingredients between the 2 mugs (i.e., 1/3 cup almond flour, 1/2 teaspoon baking powder, 1/2 teaspoon salt, 1 egg, and 2.5 Tablespoons coconut oil in each mug). Mix well.
5. Microwave each mug for 90 seconds on high. Wait a few minutes before popping them out of the mug. Slice each bread into 4 slices and use as burger buns. (Gently fry them for a few seconds in the frying pan without oil for a toasted taste.)

6. Serve the burgers (1 mini burger for each person) with the mustard, lettuce leaves, and pickles.

Nutritional Data (estimates) - per serving:

Calories: 553 Fat: 52 g Net Carbohydrates: 1 g Protein: 21 g

SPAGHETTI BOLOGNESE BAKE

Prep Time: 15 minutes

Cook Time: 45 minutes

Total Time: 60 minutes

Yield: 8 servings

2 lbs (900 g) ground beef

1/2 onion, diced

1/4 cup (60 ml) avocado oil, to cook with

Salt and pepper, to taste

1 can (400 g) diced tomatoes

1/2 can (200 g) tomato sauce

3 cloves of garlic, finely diced or minced

2 zucchinis, spiralized, shredded, or peeled into long noodle-like strands

1/2 cup (16 g) fresh basil leaves, finely chopped

1. Preheat oven to 350 F (175 C).
2. Add the avocado oil to a hot pan and brown the beef and onions.
3. Add into a large baking dish with the rest of the ingredients (except the zucchinis and basil).
4. Bake for 30 minutes.
5. Then carefully stir in the zucchini noodles and basil, let sit for 5 minutes, and serve.

Nutritional Data (estimates) - per serving:

Calories: 392 Fat: 31 g Net Carbohydrates: 5 g Protein: 20 g

MUSTARD GROUND BEEF SAUTE

Prep Time: 5 minutes

Cook Time: 15 minutes

Total Time: 20 minutes

Yield: 2 servings

0.8 lbs (360 g) ground beef

5 celery stalks, cut into thin slices

10 cherry tomatoes, halved (or 1 tomato, chopped)

1 egg

1.5 Tablespoons (20 g) yellow mustard

6 cloves of garlic, minced

Salt to taste

1 tablespoon (15 ml) coconut oil to cook with

1. Melt the coconut oil in a large frying pan or saucepan on medium heat and cook the ground beef until all of it turns brown. Stir regularly to get it to cook evenly and to break up any large chunks.
2. Add in the celery slices and cherry tomato halves and cook for 5 minutes while stirring regularly.
3. Break an egg into the pan and stir to mix it into the ground beef mixture.
4. Add in the mustard and garlic, and cook until the pieces of eggs are cooked (not liquid anymore).
5. Add salt, to taste.

Nutritional Data (estimates) - per serving:

Calories: 480 Fat: 30 g Net Carbohydrates: 6 g Protein: 40 g

GUACAMOLE BURGERS

Prep Time: 10 minutes

Cook Time: 20 minutes

Total Time: 30 minutes

Yield: 4 servings

1-1.5 lbs (454-731 g) ground beef

4 eggs

Coconut oil to cook with

1 cup (220 g) guacamole

1. With your hands, mold the ground beef into 4 patties.
2. Cook the 4 burger patties, either in a skillet with a bit of coconut oil or on a grill.
3. Once the burgers are cooked through, place to the side.
4. Fry the eggs (preferably in coconut oil) in a skillet.
5. Place 1 fried egg on top of each burger and then top with guacamole.

Nutritional Data (estimates) - per serving:

Calories: 600 Fat: 45 g Net Carbohydrates: 4 g Protein: 45 g

PRESSURE COOKER PORK SHOULDER

Prep Time: 10 minutes

Cook Time: 1 hour

Total Time: 1 hour 10 minutes

Yield: 2 servings

1 lb (454 g) pork shoulder

1 onion, diced

1 tablespoon (5 g) fresh ginger, grated

2 tablespoons (30 ml) apple cider vinegar

1 tablespoon (15 g) salt

1 teaspoon (1 g) black pepper

1 cup (240 ml) water

1. Place all the ingredients into a pressure cooker.
2. Press the Meat/Stew button (normal pressure) and then set the timer for 40 minutes. (The pressure cooker takes a few minutes of prep to get ready and then a few minutes to bring the pressure down, so the total cook time is closer to 1 hour.)

Nutritional Data (estimates) - per serving:

Calories: 550 Fat: 41 g Net Carbohydrates: 1 g Protein: 40 g

PORK AND CASHEW STIR-FRY

Prep Time: 5 minutes

Cook Time: 10 minutes

Total Time: 15 minutes

Yield: 2 servings

1/2 lb (225 g) pork tenderloin, sliced thin

1 egg, whisked

1 bell pepper, diced

1 green onion, diced

1/3 cup (40 g) cashews

1 Tablespoon (5 g) fresh ginger, grated

3 cloves of garlic, minced

1 teaspoon (5 ml) Chinese chili oil (optional)

1 Tablespoon (15 ml) sesame oil (optional)

2 Tablespoons (30 ml) tamari sauce

Salt to taste

Avocado oil to cook with

1. Place the avocado oil into a frying pan and cook the whisked egg. Place it aside on a plate.
2. Add additional avocado oil into the frying pan and cook the pork. Then add in the pepper, onion, and cashews. Saute until the pork is fully cooked, then add back in the cooked egg. Then add in the ginger, garlic, chili oil, sesame oil, tamari sauce, and salt to taste.

Nutritional Data (estimates) - per serving:

Calories: 440 Fat: 31 g Net Carbohydrates: 8 g Protein: 32 g

SPICY DRY RUB RIBS

Prep Time: 5 minutes

Cook Time: 2 hours

Total Time: 2 hours 5 minutes

Yield: 2 servings

2 lb (908 g) pork spare ribs

1 Tablespoon (15 g) salt

2 Tablespoons (12 g) paprika

1 Tablespoon (10 g) garlic powder

1 Tablespoon (7 g) onion powder

1/2 teaspoon (1 g) chili powder or cayenne pepper

1. Cut the ribs so that they're in slabs of approx. 4 ribs.
2. Place the ribs in a pot of water (make sure the ribs are submerged in the water) and boil for 1 hour (again, keep the water for broths later). (This is an easy method for cooking tender ribs - there are more complicated methods, but this is the most fool-proof one I've found.)
3. Preheat oven to 325 F (160 C).
4. Mix together the salt, paprika, garlic powder, onion powder, and cayenne pepper to form the rub. Taste the rub to see if you want to add in more of any of the spices.
5. Dip each set of ribs into the rub and place in a baking pan. Place foil over the baking pan and bake for 40 minutes. Remove the foil and bake for another 20 minutes.

Nutritional Data (estimates) - per serving:

Calories: 520 Fat: 45 g Net Carbohydrates: 2 g Protein: 25 g

CHINESE PORK SPARE RIBS

Prep Time: 10 minutes

Cook Time: 1 hour 20 minutes

Total Time: 1 hour 30 minutes

Yield: 4 servings

4 lb (1.8 kg) pork spare ribs (or back ribs), chopped into individual ribs

3 star anise

20 Szechuan peppercorns

2 Tablespoons (30 g) salt (optional)

3 cloves of garlic, minced

1/4-inch (1.25 cm) chunk of fresh ginger, grated

1/4 cup (17 g) scallions (spring onion, diced), divided into 2 parts

4 Tablespoons (60 ml) tamari sauce

2 Tablespoons (30 ml) coconut oil

1. Place the ribs in a large stockpot filled with water so that the ribs are covered.
2. After the water starts boiling, skim off any foam that forms on the top of the broth.
3. Add star anise, Szechuan peppercorns, and salt to the pot and simmer until the meat is cooked and soft (approx. 45 minutes).
4. Remove the ribs from the pot but keep the broth (pour it through a sieve to remove all solids). The broth (by itself) is wonderful to drink with just a bit of salt, or else you can use it as the base for soups.
5. In a small bowl, mix together the grated ginger, scallions, minced garlic, tamari sauce, and coconut oil.
6. Heat up a skillet (or wok if you have one) on high heat and add the ribs in batches to it. Divide the mixture so that you will have enough for each batch of ribs. Coat each batch of ribs on both sides with the mixture. Double the mixture if you prefer more sauce on the ribs.
7. Sauté the ribs on high heat until they brown and no more liquid remains in the skillet.

Nutritional Data (estimates) - per serving:

Calories: 520 Fat: 45 g Net Carbohydrates: 2 g Protein: 25 g

MU SHU PORK

Prep Time: 15 minutes

Cook Time: 15 minutes

Total Time: 30 minutes

Yield: 2 servings

1/2 lb (225 g) pork tenderloin, cut into small thin 1-inch long strips

3 eggs, whisked

15 Napa cabbage leaves, chopped into thin strips

1 cup (89 g) shiitake mushrooms, sliced

1 8-ounce (227 g) can of sliced bamboo shoots or asparagus

1/2 teaspoon (1 g) fresh ginger, grated

1 Tablespoon (15 ml) tamari sauce

1/2 teaspoon (2.5 ml) apple cider vinegar

Salt to taste

1 tablespoon + 1 teaspoon (18 ml total) coconut oil to cook in

1/4 cup (17 g) scallions (for garnish)

Lettuce leaves to serve pork in (optional)

1. Add 1 Tablespoon (15 ml) of coconut oil to a skillet on medium heat.
2. Add a little bit of salt to the whisked eggs and pour the mixture into the skillet. Let it cook undisturbed into a pancake. Flip the egg pancake once it's cooked most of the way through (it needs to be fairly solid when you flip it). Cook for a few more minutes, then place on a cutting board and cut into thin 1- inch long strips.
3. Cook the pork in a teaspoon of coconut oil. Stir with a spatula to make sure the strips don't clump together.
4. Once the pork is cooked, add in the strips of eggs, sliced mushrooms, sliced Napa cabbage, and bamboo shoots. Add in the ginger, tamari sauce, and apple cider vinegar.
5. Cook until the cabbage and mushrooms are soft. Then add salt to taste.
6. Sprinkle the scallions on top for garnish and serve dish in lettuce cups or by itself.

Nutritional Data (estimates) - per serving:

Calories: 340 Fat: 18 g Net Carbohydrates: 7 g Protein: 35 g

7. SIDE DISHES

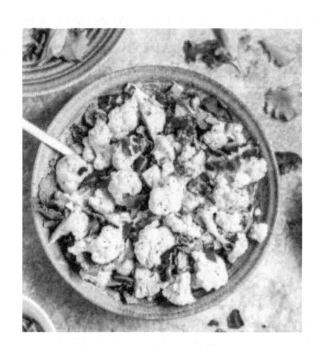

CAULIFLOWER WHITE RICE

Prep Time: 10 minutes

Cook Time: 15 minutes

Total Time: 25 minutes

Yield: 2 servings

1/2 head (approx. 220 g) of cauliflower, chopped into small florets

1 Tablespoon (15 ml) coconut oil

1. Process the cauliflower in the food processor until it forms very small "rice"- like pieces. Squeeze out excess water.
2. Add 1 Tablespoon of coconut oil into a large pot. Add in the cauliflower and let it cook on a medium heat. Stir regularly to make sure it doesn't burn. Cook until tender but not mushy.

Nutritional Data (estimates) - per serving:

Calories: 90 Fat: 7 g Net Carbohydrates: 4 g Protein: 3 g

GARLIC ZUCCHINI SAUTE

Prep Time: 5 minutes

Cook Time: 12 minutes

Total Time: 17 minutes

Yield: 4 servings

2 lb (908 g) zucchini, chopped into small pieces or slices

6 cloves of garlic, minced

Olive oil to saute in

1. Add olive oil into a skillet on medium heat. Add in the zucchini and saute until they're softened (approx. 10 minutes). Add the garlic and saute for 1-2 minutes more.

Nutritional Data (estimates) - per serving:

Calories: 70 Fat: 4 g Net Carbohydrates: 4 g Protein: 0 g

MICROWAVE QUICK BREAD

Prep Time: 3.5 minutes

Cook Time: 1.5 minutes

Total Time: 5 minutes

Yield: 2 servings

1/3 cup (35 g) almond flour

1/2 teaspoon (2 g) baking powder

1 egg, whisked

2.5 Tablespoons (37 ml) ghee or coconut oil, melted

1. Grease a mug and mix all the ingredients in it with a fork.
2. Microwave for 90 seconds on high. (You may need to adjust the time for your microwave settings.)
3. Cool for a few minutes, pop out of mug gently and slice into 4 thin slices.

Nutritional Data (estimates) - per serving:

Calories: 260 Fat: 26 g Net Carbohydrates: 2 g Protein: 6 g

CREAMY CAULIFLOWER MASH

Prep Time: 10 minutes

Cook Time: 10 minutes

Total Time: 20 minutes

Yield: 2 servings

1/2 head of cauliflower (approx. 220 g), broken into small florets

2 Tablespoons (30 ml) ghee (or coconut oil)

1/4 cup (60 ml) coconut milk, from a can shaken & at room temp

Salt to taste

1. Place the cauliflower florets into a large microwaveable bowl with 1/4 cup of water at the bottom. Microwave on high until they are softened (around 10-12 minutes). Check every 3 minutes to make sure there's water in the bowl still. Alternatively, you can steam the cauliflower florets in a steamer.
2. Blend the cauliflower with ghee, coconut milk, and salt until smooth.

Nutritional Data (estimates) - per serving:

Calories: 200 Fat: 20 g Net Carbohydrates: 4 g Protein: 4 g

SPINACH ALMOND SAUTE

Prep Time: 0 minutes

Cook Time: 10 minutes

Total Time: 10 minutes

Yield: 2 servings

1 lb (454 g) spinach leaves

3 Tablespoons (12 g) almond slices

Salt to taste

1 Tablespoon (15 ml) avocado oil for cooking

1. Place the 1 Tablespoon of avocado oil into a large pot on medium heat.
2. Add in the spinach and let it cook down.
3. Once the spinach is cooked down, add the salt to taste and stir.
4. Before serving, stir in the almond slices.

Nutritional Data (estimates) - per serving:

Calories: 150 Fat: 11 g Net Carbohydrates: 4 g Protein: 8 g

EASY BACON BRUSSELS SPROUTS

Prep Time: 5 minutes

Cook Time: 20 minutes

Total Time: 25 minutes

Yield: 6 servings

2 lbs (908 g) Brussels sprouts

1 lb (454 g) bacon, uncooked

1. Boil the Brussels sprouts for 10 minutes until tender.
2. While the Brussels sprouts are boiling, chop the bacon into small pieces (approx. 1/2-inch wide), and cook the bacon pieces in a large pot on medium heat. When the bacon is crispy, add in the drained Brussels sprouts.
3. Cook for 10 more minutes on high heat, stirring occasionally to make sure nothing gets burnt on the bottom of the pan.

Nutritional Data (estimates) - per serving:

Calories: 400 Fat: 35 g Net Carbohydrates: 6 g Protein: 14 g

TURMERIC CAULIFLOWER PANCAKES

Prep Time: 10 minutes

Cook Time: 40 minutes

Total Time: 50 minutes

Yield: 8 servings

1 head of cauliflower, broken into florets

2 eggs, whisked

1 cup (120 g) almond flour

2 Tablespoons (12 g) turmeric powder

2 cloves of garlic, peeled and minced

1 Tablespoon (15 ml) coconut oil, for greasing the baking tray

Salt and pepper, to taste

1. Preheat oven to 350 F (175 C).
2. Steam the cauliflower florets until softened.
3. Mash the cauliflower and mix with the eggs, almond flour, turmeric, and garlic. Season with salt and pepper.
4. Form 8 flat patties. Place on a greased baking tray and bake for 30 minutes until slightly browned.

Nutritional Data (estimates) - per serving:

Calories: 123 Fat: 9 g Net Carbohydrates: 3 g Protein: 5 g

TANGY RED CABBAGE COLESLAW

Prep Time: 10 minutes

Cook Time: 0 minutes

Total Time: 10 minutes

Yield: 4 servings

2 cups of shredded red cabbage (approx 1/4 head of cabbage)

1/4 red onion, sliced

1/4 cup (20 g) walnuts, chopped

2 Tablespoons (30 ml) lemon juice

1/4 cup (60 ml) mayo

1 teaspoon (5 ml) mustard

1. Toss all the ingredients together well and enjoy.

Nutritional Data (estimates) - per serving:

Calories: 164 Fat: 17 g Net Carbohydrates: 3 g Protein: 2 g

CAULIFLOWER NOTATO SALAD

Prep Time: 5 minutes

Cook Time: 10 minutes

Total Time: 15 minutes

Yield: 4 servings

1 head of cauliflower, broken into florets

2 Tablespoons of chives, finely diced

1/4 cup (60 ml) mayo

2 teaspoons (10 ml) mustard

Salt and pepper to taste

1. Boil or steam the cauliflower florets until tender. Run immediately under cold water to cool. Then drain well.
2. Toss the florets with the chives, mayo, mustard, and salt and pepper.

Nutritional Data (estimates) - per serving:

Calories: 136 Fat: 12 g Net Carbohydrates: 4 g Protein: 3 g

ROASTED CAULIFLOWER

Prep Time: 15 minutes

Cook Time: 1 hour 15 minutes

Total Time: 1 hour 30 minutes

Yield: 4 servings

Half of a large cauliflower (approx. 220 g), broken into florets

2 teaspoons (4 g) turmeric powder or garlic powder or Italian seasoning

2 teaspoons (10 g) salt

2 Tablespoons (30 ml) olive oil

1. Preheat oven to 350 F (175 C).
2. Mix the cauliflower florets with the spice/herb, salt, and olive oil.
3. Spread the florets out in a baking tray and bake covered with foil for 75 minutes.

Nutritional Data (estimates) - per serving:

Calories: 90 Fat: 7 g Net Carbohydrates: 3 g Protein: 0 g

8.

CONDIMENTS, SEASONING & SAUCES

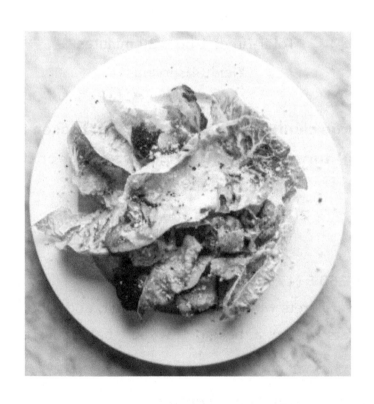

COCONUT MAYONNAISE

Prep Time: 15 minutes

Cook Time: 0 minutes

Total Time: 15 minutes

Yield: approx. 1.5 cups

2 egg yolks

2 Tablespoons (30 ml) of apple cider vinegar

1 cup (240 ml) coconut oil, melted (but not too hot)

1. Blend or whisk the 2 egg yolks with the 2 Tablespoons (30 ml) of apple cider vinegar.
2. Slowly add in the coconut oil while blending (I used a blender and added in the coconut oil from the hole at top of the blender approximately 1/2 tablespoon at a time until it forms a mayo texture).
3. Add in rest of the oil (and a bit more if you want a less thick texture) and blend well.
4. Use immediately (if you want to store it in the fridge, then use 1/2 cup olive oil or avocado oil and 1/2 cup coconut oil instead of only coconut oil, as the coconut oil will make the mayo solidify in the fridge. We try to use it within a week.)

SUBSTITUTIONS

- Olive oil or avocado oil can be used instead of coconut oil.
- Spices and herbs can be added for different types of mayo.
- Lemon juice can be used instead of apple cider vinegar (but it gives a different taste to the mayo).

Nutritional Data (estimates) - per tablespoon:

Calories: 80 Fat: 9 g Net Carbohydrates: 0 g Protein: 0 g

CASHEW CHEESE

Prep Time: 10 minutes

Cook Time: 0 minutes

Total Time: 10 minutes

Yield: 1 cup

1/2 cup (70 g) raw cashews, soaked overnight

1 Tablespoon (15 ml) coconut oil

1/2 cup (120 ml) water

1. Place the raw cashews into a bowl of room temperature water so that it covers the cashews, drape a paper towel or tea towel over the bowl to prevent dust settling, and soak overnight.
2. Blend the soaked cashews, 1/2 cup fresh water, and coconut oil until smooth.

Nutritional Data (estimates) - per tablespoon:

Calories: 32 Fat: 3 g Net Carbohydrates: 1 g Protein: 1 g

CAESAR DRESSING

Prep Time: 15 minutes

Cook Time: 0 minutes

Total Time: 15 minutes

Yield: approx. 1.5 cups

2 egg yolks

1/4 cup (60 ml) apple cider vinegar

1 cup (240 ml) coconut oil, melted

6 anchovies

2 teaspoons (9 g) Dijon mustard

2 large cloves of garlic, minced

1/4 teaspoon (1 g) salt

1/4 teaspoon (1 g) freshly ground black pepper

1. Blend or whisk the 2 egg yolks with the apple cider vinegar.
2. Slowly add in the coconut oil while blending until it forms a mayo texture.
3. Add in rest of the oil, the anchovies, mustard, garlic, salt, and pepper and blend well.

Nutritional Data (estimates) - per tablespoon:

Calories: 80 Fat: 9 g Net Carbohydrates:0g Protein: 0g

COCONUT RANCH DRESSING

Prep Time: 10 minutes

Cook Time: 0 minutes

Total Time: 10 minutes

Yield: approx. 1/2 cup

1/4 cup (60 ml) of mayo (see page 125 for recipe)

1/4 cup (60 ml) coconut milk

1 clove of garlic, minced

1/2 teaspoon (1 g) onion powder

1 Tablespoon (4 g) fresh parsley, finely chopped (or 1 tsp (0.5 g) dried parsley)

1 Tablespoon (3 g) fresh chives, finely chopped (or omit)

1 teaspoon (1 g) fresh dill, finely chopped (or 1/2 tsp (0.5 g) dried dill)

Dash of salt

Dash of pepper

1. Mix together the mayo, coconut milk, onion powder, salt, and pepper with a fork.
2. Gently mix in the garlic and fresh herbs.

Nutritional Data (estimates) - per tablespoon:

Calories: 50 Fat: 6 g Net Carbohydrates: 0g Protein:0g

HOMEMADE ITALIAN SEASONING

Prep Time: 5 minutes

Cook Time: 0 minutes

Total Time: 5 minutes

Yield: 1 cup

1/4 cup (12 g) dried basil

1/4 cup (12 g) dried rosemary

1/4 cup (12 g) dried thyme

1/4 cup (12 g) dried oregano

1 Tablespoon (10 g) garlic powder

1 Tablespoon (7 g) onion powder

1. Mix all the ingredients together well and store in an airtight container.

Nutritional Data (estimates) - per tablespoon:

Calories: 10 Fat: 0 g Net Carbohydrates:1g Protein: 0g

CAJUN SEASONING

Prep Time: 5 minutes

Cook Time: 0 minutes

Total Time: 5 minutes

Yield: 6 Tablespoons

1.5 Tablespoons (10 g) paprika

1.5 Tablespoons (15 g) garlic powder

1/2 Tablespoon (3 g) onion powder

1/2 Tablespoon (2 g) black pepper

1 teaspoon (2 g) cayenne pepper

1 teaspoon (2 g) dried oregano

1 teaspoon (1 g) dried thyme

1 teaspoon (1 g) dried basil

1-2 teaspoons (5-10 g) of salt (to taste)

1. Mix all the dried spices and herbs together and store in an airtight jar.

Nutritional Data (estimates) - per tablespoon:

Calories: 15 Fat: 0g Net Carbohydrates: 2g Protein: 0g

SLOW COOKER GHEE

Prep Time: 0 minutes

Cook Time: 3 hours

Total Time: 3 hours

Yield: 2 cups

16 oz (454 g) butter

1. Place butter into slow cooker and place lid on (slightly ajar so that steam escapes).
2. Turn slow cooker on low for 2-3 hours until milk solids brown and fall to bottom.
3. Strain through a cheesecloth into glass jars to store.

Nutritional Data (estimates) - per tablespoon:

Calories: 120 Fat: 14 g Net Carbohydrates: 0 g Protein: 0 g

COCONUT BUTTER

Prep Time: 10 minutes

Cook Time: 0 minutes

Total Time: 10 minutes

Yield: approx. 3 cups

6 cups (480 g) of unsweetened shredded coconut (or coconut flakes or coconut powder)

2 Tablespoons (15 ml) coconut oil, melted (if not using the VitaMix with a tamper or a Blendtec with the twister jar)

1. Add the shredded coconut to the blender or food processor and blend on high.
2. If using the VitaMix with a tamper or a Blendtec with the twister jar, push the coconut down while you blend. Otherwise, stop the blender and push the coconut down with a spoon, and repeat 3 times.

3. If not using a VitaMix or a Blendtec, add the melted coconut oil in and blend on high for 10 minutes.

Nutritional Data (estimates) - per tablespoon:

Calories: 60 Fat: 6g Net Carbohydrates: 1g Protein: 1g

GARLIC SAUCE

Prep Time: 5 minutes

Cook Time: 0 minutes

Total Time: 5 minutes

Yield: approx. 1.5 cups

1 head garlic, peeled

1 teaspoon (5 g) salt

Approx. 1/4 cup (60 ml) lemon juice

Approx. 1 cup (240 ml) olive oil

1. Place the garlic cloves and salt into the blender. Then add in around 1/8 cup of the lemon juice and 1/2 cup of olive oil.
2. Blend well for 5-10 seconds, then slow your blender down and drizzle in more lemon juice and olive oil alternately until a creamy consistency forms.

Nutritional Data (estimates) - per tablespoon:

Calories: 80 Fat: 9g Net Carbohydrates: 0g Protein: 0g

EASY GUACAMOLE

Prep Time: 10 minutes

Cook Time: 0 minutes

Total Time: 10 minutes

Yield: 1 cup

2 ripe avocados, flesh scooped out

1 small tomato, diced

1/4 cup (8 g) cilantro, finely chopped

Juice from half a lime

Salt to taste

1 jalapeño, finely chopped (optional)

1/2 teaspoon (1 g) chili powder (optional)

1 teaspoon (3 g) garlic powder (optional)

1 teaspoon (2g) onion powder (optional)

1. Mash up the avocado flesh using a spoon or fork. Mix in the other ingredients.

Nutritional Data (estimates) - per tablespoon:

Calories: 40 Fat: 4g Net Carbohydrates: 1g Protein: 1g

9. SNACKS

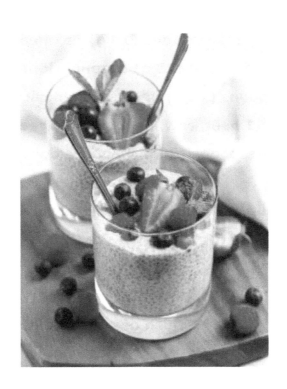

RED VELVET COOKIES

Prep Time: 15 minutes

Cook Time: 15 minutes

Total Time: 30 minutes

Yield: 8 servings

2 cups (240 g) almond flour

2 Tablespoons (14 g) flaxmeal

1/4 cup (28 g) coconut flour

3 Tablespoons (18 g) unsweetened cacao powder

1 beet, raw, peeled and diced

2 Tablespoons (30 ml) apple cider vinegar

1/3 cup (80 ml) ghee

1/3-1/2 cup erythritol (or Keto sweetener, to taste)

1 egg, whisked

1/2 teaspoon (1 g) baking soda

1 teaspoon (5 ml) vanilla extract

Dash of salt

1. Preheat oven to 350 F (175 C).
2. Puree the beet and add in the vinegar and ghee.
3. Mix all the cookie ingredients together in a bowl until a soft dough forms.
4. Form small balls from the dough (use a Tablespoon scoop). Press into a round cookie and place onto a parchment paper lined baking tray. The cookies will spread so make sure to leave enough room between the cookies. Makes around 24 small cookies.
5. Bake for 12-15 minutes. Let cool before enjoying.

Nutritional Data (estimates) - per serving:

Calories: 227 Fat: 25 g Net Carbohydrates: 3 g Protein: 7 g

CHOCOLATE COFFEE COCONUT TRUFFLES

Prep Time: 10 minutes

Cook Time: 5 hours set time

Total Time: 10 minutes + 5 hours

Yield: 6 servings

1/2 cup (120 g) coconut butter (see page 130 for recipe), melted

3 Tablespoons (15 g) 100% cacao powder

1 Tablespoon (5 g) ground coffee beans

1 Tablespoon (5 g) unsweetened coconut flakes

Dash of stevia (optional)

1 Tablespoon (15 ml) coconut oil, melted

1. Mix all the ingredients together and pour into an ice-cube tray or muffin cups.
2. Freeze for 4-5 hours. Defrost at room temperature for 15-20 minutes before serving.

Nutritional Data (estimates) - per serving:

Calories: 160 Fat: 15g Net Carbohydrates: 3g Protein: 2g

CHOCOLATE CHIA PUDDING

Prep Time: 5 minutes

Cook Time: 8 hours set time

Total Time: 5 minutes + 8 hrs

Yield: 2 servings

2 Tablespoons (10 g) unsweetened cacao powder

1 cup (240 ml) unsweetened coconut milk

1/3 cup (215 g) chia seeds

1 Tablespoon (5 g) unsweetened shredded coconut (for topping)

Spices and/or sweetener of choice

1. Mix together all the ingredients (except the shredded coconut) in a bowl and refrigerate overnight.
2. Blend the mixture until smooth. Pour into cups and top with shredded coconut.

Nutritional Data (estimates) - per serving:

Calories: 300 Fat: 24 g Net Carbohydrates: 3 g Protein: 8 g

BLACK & WHITE LAYERED PEPPERMINT PATTIES

Prep Time: 15 minutes

Cook Time: 3 hours set time

Total Time: 15 minutes + 3 hrs

Yield: 12 servings

For the white layers:

½ cup (120 g) coconut butter

¼ cup (20 g) unsweetened shredded coconut

2 Tablespoons (30 ml) coconut oil

1 teaspoon (5 ml) peppermint extract (add more to taste)

Erythritol and stevia, to taste (optional)

For the black layers:

4 oz (115 g) 100% dark chocolate

4 Tablespoons (60 ml) coconut oil

1. To make the white layers, soften the coconut butter and the 2 tablespoons of coconut oil and mix them together with the unsweetened shredded coconut, sweetener, and peppermint extract.
2. Spoon 2 teaspoons of the white mixture into each mini muffin cup and refrigerate for 1 hour to set. Check this layer is solid before proceeding to the next step. If you don't have a mini muffin tray, then use a regular muffin tray - serving size will be half of a patty.
3. To make the black layers, melt the 4 tablespoons of coconut oil and the 4 oz dark chocolate and combine together well. Spoon 1 teaspoon of the black mixture into each mini muffin cup so that it forms a thin layer above the already solid white layer. Set in fridge for 1 hour. Check this layer is solid before going to the next step.
4. Repeat steps 2 and 3 for as many layers as you want.

Nutritional Data (estimates) - per serving:

Calories: 100 Fat: 10 g Net Carbohydrates: 2 g Protein: 1 g

SAVORY ITALIAN CRACKERS

Prep Time: 15 minutes

Cook Time: 10 minutes

Total Time: 25 minutes

Yield: 4 servings

1.5 cups (165 g) almond flour

1 egg

2 Tablespoons (30 ml) olive oil

3/4 teaspoon (4 g) salt

1/4 teaspoon (0.5 g) basil

1/2 teaspoon (1 g) thyme

1/4 teaspoon (0.5 g) oregano

1/2 teaspoon (1 g) onion powder

1/4 teaspoon (0.5 g) garlic powder

1. Preheat oven to 350 F (175 C).
2. Mix all the ingredients well to form a dough.
3. Shape dough into a long rectangular log (use some foil or cling film to pack the dough tight) and then cut into thin slices (approximately 0.2 inches (0.5 cm) thick). Gently place each slice onto a parchment paper-lined baking tray. It makes approx. 20-30 crackers, depending on size.
4. Bake for 10-12 minutes.

Nutritional Data (estimates) - per serving:

Calories: 280 Fat: 25g Net Carbohydrates: 3g Protein: 9g

CHOCOLATE CASHEW ICE CREAM

Prep Time: 10 minutes

Cook Time: varies, for making cashew cheese and freezing ice cream

Total Time: varies

Yield: 6 servings

1 cup (240 ml) cashew cheese

1/4 cup (60 ml) coconut cream

1 oz (28 g) 100% dark chocolate, melted

Erythritol and stevia, to taste

1. Blend all the ingredients together really well.
2. Pour into a container and freeze.
3. Best enjoyed after 1-2 hours. If you freeze it for longer, then you'll need to defrost it first to soften it before enjoying.

Nutritional Data (estimates) - per serving:

Calories: 131 Fat: 11g Net Carbohydrates: 3g Protein: 3g

CHOCOLATE COVERED PECANS

Prep Time: 5 min

Cook Time: 25 min + 2 hrs set time

Total Time: 30 min + 2 hrs

Yield: 4 servings

40-45 pecan halves (approx. 2.5 oz)

2 oz (56 g) 100% dark chocolate

Spices of your choosing - my favorites were cinnamon, nutmeg, and salt

1. Preheat oven to 350 F (175 C).
2. Place the pecan halves in a single layer on parchment paper. Bake for 7 minutes.
3. Let them cool. Meanwhile, melt the dark chocolate.
4. Dip each pecan half in the melted chocolate with a fork and place back on the parchment paper. Sprinkle spice on top. Refrigerate for 1-2 hours to set.

Nutritional Data (estimates) - per serving:

Calories: 160 Fat: 15 g Net Carbohydrates: 5 g Protein: 3 g

CARROT CUPCAKES WITH CASHEW CHEESE FROSTING

Prep Time: 15 minutes

Cook Time: 30 minutes

Total Time: 45 minutes

Yield: 16 servings

For the cupcakes:

3 eggs, whisked

1/2 cup erythritol (or to taste)

2 carrots (150 g), shredded (squeeze out as much of the liquid as possible)

2 teaspoons (10 ml) vanilla extract

1 cup (120 g) almond flour

2 Tablespoons (14 g) flaxmeal

1/4 cup (20 g) shredded coconut

1/2 cup (59 g) walnuts, chopped

3/4 cup (180 ml) ghee or coconut oil

2 teaspoons (9 g) baking powder

1/2 teaspoon (2 g) baking soda

2 teaspoons (4 g) cinnamon powder

1 teaspoon (2 g) ginger powder

1 tablespoon (15 ml) apple cider vinegar

Dash of nutmeg

Dash of salt

For the frosting:

1/4 cup (60 ml) cashew cheese

2 Tablespoons (30 ml) coconut cream

2 Tablespoons (30 ml) coconut oil

Erythritol or stevia, to taste

1/2 teaspoon (3 ml) vanilla extract

Dash of salt

For the topping:

Small handful of chopped walnuts and shredded carrot

1. Preheat oven to 350 F (175 C).
2. Mix all the cupcake ingredients together.
3. Pour into a cupcake pan (makes approx. 12 cupcakes) and bake for 30 minutes.

4. Meanwhile make the frosting by blending all the ingredients together (don't melt any of the ingredients - just keep them at room temperature and blend them and if it gets too liquidy, then refrigerate them for a bit to let it solidify more). Spread on top of the cupcakes once they're cooled. Top with leftover chopped walnuts and shredded carrots.

Nutritional Data (estimates) - per serving:

Calories: 210 Fat: 21g Net Carbohydrates: 2g Protein: 4g

10. DRINKS AND BROTHS

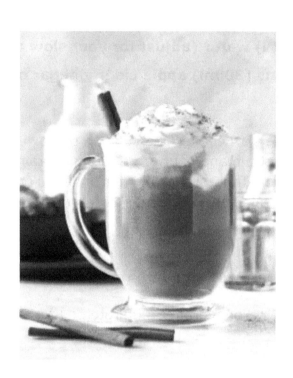

EASY BONE BROTH

Prep Time: 5 minutes

Cook Time: 10 hours

Total Time: 10 hours 5 minutes

Yield: 8-16 servings

3-4 lbs (1.5-2 kg) of bones (I typically use beef bones)

1 gallon (4 l) water (adjust for your slow cooker size)

2 Tablespoons (30 ml) apple cider vinegar or lemon juice

1. Add everything to the slow cooker and cook on the low setting for 10 hours.
2. Cool the broth, then strain and pour broth into a container.
3. Store the broth in the refrigerator or freezer until you're ready to use it.
4. Scoop out the congealed fat on top of the broth (optional, but the broth is otherwise very fatty).
5. Heat broth when needed (with spices, vegetables, etc).

Nutritional Data (estimates) - per serving:

Calories: 80 Fat: 2g Net Carbohydrates: 0g Protein: 12g

COCONUT MASALA CHAI

Prep Time: 5 minutes

Cook Time: 5 minutes

Total Time: 10 minutes

Yield: 2 servings

1 cup (240 ml) coconut milk

1 cup (240 ml) water

Stevia to taste (optional)

1 Tablespoon (2 g) loose black tea leaves

Pinch of masala tea spice blend (recipe below)

Masala tea spice blend:

1 Tablespoon (7 g) nutmeg

1 Tablespoon (5 g) ginger powder

1 Tablespoon (6g) cardamom

1 Tablespoon (5 g) black pepper

1 Tablespoon (8 g) cinnamon

1 teaspoon (2 g) cloves

1 Tablespoon (5 g) dried basil (optional), ground into a powder

1. Heat the coconut milk and water in a saucepan.
2. Add in the stevia, the tea, and the spice blend. Mix well.
3. Heat at a low simmer for approx. 4-5 minutes.
4. Taste the tea and add more sweetener or spices to taste.
5. Pour through a strainer (to remove the tea leaves) and serve immediately.

Nutritional Data (estimates) - per serving:

Calories: 300 Fat: 30g Net Carbohydrates: 2g Protein: 3g

GINGER BASIL TEA

Prep Time: 5 minutes

Cook Time: 0 minutes

Total Time: 5 minutes

Yield: 2 servings

2 cups (480 ml) boiling water

1/2 teaspoon (1 g) fresh ginger, grated (or 10 very thin slices of ginger)

4 fresh basil leaves

1. Add the ginger and basil to a cup or teapot and pour boiling water into the cup/teapot.
2. Brew for 5 minutes. Enjoy hot or cold.

Nutritional Data (estimates) - per serving:

Calories: 0 Fat: 0g Net Carbohydrates: 0g Protein: 0g

PUMPKIN SPICE LATTE

Total Time: 5 minutes

Yield: 1 cup of coffee

1 cup (240 ml) black coffee

1 Tablespoon (15 g) pumpkin puree

1/4 teaspoon (1 g) cinnamon

1/4 teaspoon (1 g) nutmeg

Dash of cloves

1 Tablespoon (15 ml) ghee

1. Place all the ingredients into a blender and blend well for 15 seconds.

Nutritional Data (estimates) - per serving:

Calories: 120 Fat: 13 g Net Carbohydrates: 1 g Protein: 1 g

COCONUT GHEE COFFEE

Total Time: 5 minutes

Yield: 1 cup of coffee

1/2 Tablespoon (7 g) ghee

1/2 Tablespoon (7 g) coconut oil

1-2 cups (240-480 ml) of whatever coffee you like (or black or rooibos tea)

1 Tablespoon (15 ml) almond milk or coconut milk

1. Put the ghee, coconut oil, almond milk (or coconut milk), and the coffee into a blender.
2. Blend for 5-10 seconds. The coffee turns a foamy, creamy color. Pour it into your favorite coffee cup and enjoy!
3. If you don't have a blender, then try using a milk frother.

Nutritional Data (estimates) - per serving:

Calories: 150 Fat: 15 g Net Carbohydrates: 0 g Protein: 0 g

LEMON THYME INFUSED ICED TEA

Total Time: 10 minutes + overnight infusion

Yield: 6-8 cups of tea

4-6 cups (1-1.5 l) of black tea

6 sprigs of lemon thyme or other herb or spice

1. Brew the black tea.
2. Remove the tea bag(s) and add 2 sprigs of lemon thyme into the hot tea.
3. Let cool and then refrigerate overnight.
4. Remove the lemon thyme and serve with ice and fresh sprigs of lemon thyme for decoration.

Nutritional Data (estimates) - per serving:

Calories: 0 Fat: 0 g Net Carbohydrates: 0 g Protein: 0 g

COCONUT ICED TEA LATTE

Total Time: 15 minutes

Yield: 2 cups of tea

2 cups (480 ml) black tea

3 Tablespoons (30 ml) coconut milk (or to taste)

Stevia to taste (optional)

1. Brew the black tea.
2. Add in the coconut milk and stevia to taste.
3. Blend for a few seconds or use a milk frother.
4. Let cool for 10 minutes, then pour into a glass with ice.

Nutritional Data (estimates) - per cup:

Calories: 30 Fat: 3 g Net Carbohydrates: 0g Protein:0g

About the Author

Khloe Faulkner is passionate writer about empowering people to lead active healthy lifestyles by teaching them the personalized skills they need to fuel themselves with whole foods while maintaining a healthy life balance.

Made in the USA
Las Vegas, NV
16 January 2024

84485416R00052